CAREERS IN DENTAL LABORATORY TECHNOLOGY

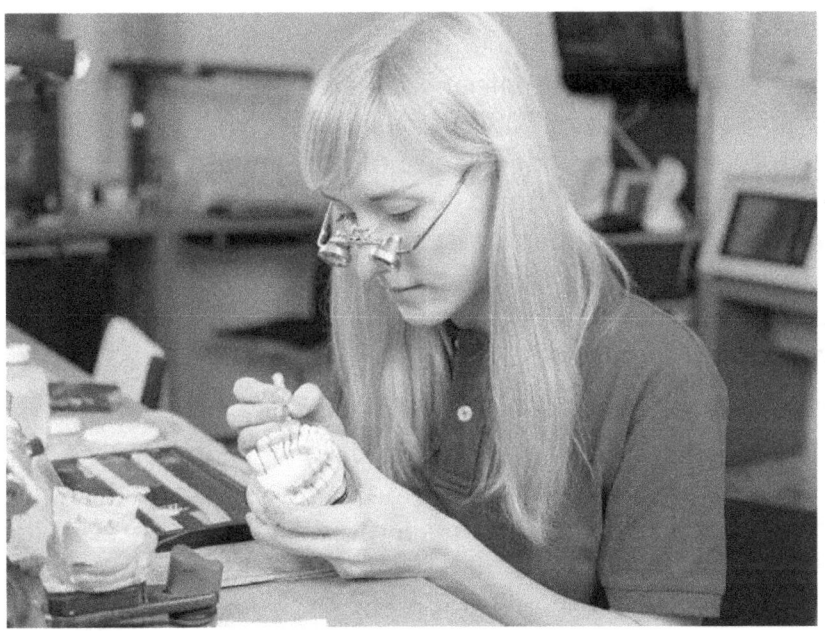

THE FIELD OF DENTAL LAB TECHNOLOGY is an ever-growing (and often overlooked) career that combines healthcare, technology and art. This is a solid opportunity for people who want to help others and be a part of ever-changing technology, and who consider themselves equal parts scientist and artist.

Dental lab technicians, also known as dental techs, work independently to recreate a patient's real smile using prosthetics in order to improve health and appearance. They handle small tools and must possess an eye for detail in order to accomplish this task. Dental laboratory technicians do not work directly with patients, but they are an important part of overall dental healthcare, providing the physical elements that allow for complete smiles and better tooth function.

Dental laboratory technicians are an extension of dentistry, which dates back to 7000 BC. It is a field with a fascinating history as it is a demonstration of humanity's evolution in terms of the technologies we use and the understanding we have of the human body and its functions. For example, the earliest cavities were thought to be caused by worms burrowing into the teeth, and the first fillings were composed of beeswax.

Over the years, the technology used in the field has developed considerably, from carving ivory and animal bones to construct false teeth, to using lasers and plastic to create brand-new smiles. It is a rewarding field because the items you make have a direct impact on the patient's health, and the results last long after you have completed the work.

In general, it takes two years to become eligible to work as a fully qualified dental laboratory technician, and once you enter the field you can be promoted to laboratory supervisor or even establish your own lab – an enticing opportunity for those who consider themselves the entrepreneurial type. When you own your own company, the salary opportunities are unlimited.

Dental laboratory technicians possess a very specific set of skills, as their job is part technology and human artistry. While machines are responsible for part of the construction, the finishing touches can only be done with a craftsman's hand, requiring incredible eye for detail, creativity and a very well developed sense of dexterity.

This field could experience major growth in the upcoming years as more and more people are becoming conscious of how they look, making it an excellent time to pursue the field. As cosmetic dentistry becomes the norm in modern day society, items like braces are in demand for fixing crooked teeth, veneers are being requested to cover stains and change the actual shape of the teeth, and crowns, dentures and implants are put in place to hide missing teeth and camouflage gaps. There could be an increasing need for dental laboratory technicians and their talents to construct all of these different dental technologies.

WHAT YOU CAN DO NOW

IF YOU WANT TO SET YOURSELF UP for a career in dental laboratory technology, there are some things you can do while you are still in high school. The first is taking art classes, particularly those that involve sculpture, shapes, and color theory. If they are not offered at your school, explore different options in your town. Community centers, local colleges, and art studios are a great place to look. Sculpture will give you a way to practice using tools to create and change pieces of existing material into a new form. That is exactly what dental laboratory technicians do with alloys, plastics, and waxes. Learning the art of shapes will prepare you to notice patterns and imperfections in the teeth of patients. Color theory can help you distinguish between small color changes. These combined skills provide the basics for constructing more accurate prosthetics for patients.

Take advantage of any opportunities to explore related technology. Enroll in computer classes, especially those involving 3D art and animation. Dental lab technicians use these programs to generate computer models of teeth that serve as the basis for patients' prosthetics. Understanding how to use this technology will make training for a career as a dental laboratory technician easier.

Develop your fine motor skills in classes like shop and technical education. Spend time grasping and using small tools to develop your hand-eye coordination and dexterity.

You may also want to practice working independently away from the distractions of a team because dental laboratory technicians tend to work in solitude on the job.

HISTORY OF THE CAREER

DENTAL LABORATORY TECHNOLOGY IS an extension of the field of dentistry, which dates back to 7000 BC in the Indus Valley Civilization (in what today is northeast Afghanistan and Pakistan). The earliest tools of the trade were bow drills used for fixing ailments, and beeswax for tooth fillings. In ancient Greece, wires were introduced to stabilize loose teeth, and the Etruscans developed dental bridges in 700 BC. Rinses of chemical and vegetable plaster were used to treat oral pain. Wooden dentures and teeth implants made of bone and ivory are also remnants of dental practices long ago.

Although knowledge of teeth was beginning to evolve, the methods remained quite primitive for centuries. For example, it was thought that worms were the cause of cavities, burrowing into your teeth and living there. Some "dentists" (who were actually more likely barbers who used their tools to extract painful teeth) even mistook patients' nerves as worms and attempted to extract them. To say that sounds painful is an understatement.

Dentistry as we know it today started sometime between 1650 and 1800. Pierre Fauchard, known as "the father of modern dentistry" made incredible advances in the field by utilizing tools from a variety of craftsmen such as watchmakers, jewelers, and barbers. He also shaped our understanding of what causes tooth decay, being the first to cite sugar as the culprit. He actually treated cavities with fillings that are very much the same as those used today.

Fauchard was also the father of dental laboratory technology, since he pioneered the field of dental prosthetics. Using things like carved pieces of bone or ivory, he would replace lost teeth. He also developed a method of straightening teeth after discovering that teeth would gradually move when attached to a guiding device. He constructed the first braces out of gold and waxed linen, and adhered them to the teeth with silk threads.

In the 1760s, British surgeon John Hunter published two important books that laid the groundwork for modern dental technology: *National History of Human Teeth* and *Practical Treatise of The Diseases of Teeth*. Hunter also began to experiment with tooth transplants, hypothesizing that in order for tooth transplants to work, donated teeth should be as fresh as possible. While the act of donating teeth did not quite catch on (and the recipients of those teeth finding that the new ones did end up falling out again after a period of time), Hunter's contributions to healthcare are the foundation of modern day organ transplants.

In the United States, George Washington was one of the first Americans to become a famous dental patient with his prosthetic teeth. The first American dental school, the Baltimore College of Dental Surgery, opened in 1840. That same year also saw the formation of the first national organization, the American Society of Dental Surgeons, along with the first dental magazine, *American Journal of Dental Science*. At the end of the 19th century, government regulation of dentistry began, controlling who could perform dental procedures and how those procedures were done. The American Dental Association (ADA) was also established.

Colgate became the first company in the US to mass produce toothpaste in 1873, with the first mass-produced toothbrush following in 1885. It is believed that toothbrushes originated in ancient China and were created from pigs' necks or wood. The first electric toothbrush was made in Switzerland in 1939. Proper tooth care was recommended in many countries around the world before it caught on in the United States. It was not until after World War II, when the soldiers came back from war, that regularly brushing teeth became commonplace in the US. Interestingly enough, Novocain is also a byproduct of war. It was invented in 1905 to anesthetize soldiers in the field. From there, it was picked up as a tool in dental care.

When the demand for more refined systems and procedures grew beyond the average dentist's capability, the outsourcing of prosthetics production in a lab began. Dr. W. H. Stowe was the first dedicated laboratory technician. He started as a dentist himself in the late 1800s, but his reputation as a skilled technician soon had him accepting orders from many dentists. It became apparent that there was a demand for this type of work, so he opened a dental laboratory in Boston in 1887. It is largely acknowledged to be the first commercial dental laboratory in America.

Stowe developed an apprenticeship training program – the first of its kind – out of necessity, because the required skills were not being taught at any school. As more and more technicians were trained, they left to open additional laboratories. For the first time in dental history, there became an obvious division between the professions of dentist and dental laboratory technician.

Edward H. Angle played an enormous part in orthodontics, developing a classification system for crooked teeth and starting the first school of orthodontics in 1901.

Two national organizations were formed to represent dental laboratory technicians. In 1950, the owners of several dental laboratories around the United States met in Chicago and agreed to create one unified group, the National Association of Dental Laboratories (NADL). Today, the group claims nearly 1,000 laboratory members nationwide.

Dental implants were successfully demonstrated in the 1950s, and Invisalign braces, the clear plastic caps that are worn to straighten teeth without wires, were introduced in 2000.

As technology becomes more advanced, dental laboratory technicians will have access to increasingly sophisticated tools and software that will permit even greater contributions to dental healthcare.

WHERE YOU WILL WORK

ALTHOUGH DENTAL LABORATORY technicians work closely with dentists, only a small number actually work in dentists' offices. Most of the time, as the job title implies, these careerists work in commercial dental laboratories that operate independently of the dentists they serve. The labs can range in size from two people up to 200 depending on the location, the demand for prosthetics in communities served, and the number of other dental laboratories nearby. However, most are small, privately owned businesses with fewer than five technicians. There are dental laboratories throughout all 50 states, which makes it a very secure and easily transferable career if you plan to move from place to place.

Some dental laboratory technicians work for hospitals providing dental services, including most notably the US Department of Veterans Affairs hospitals. A small number of technicians are self-employed and work in their own laboratories, usually as a part-time endeavor.

The work itself takes place inside a modern lab environment with approximately 40 hours of standing or sitting in a week. In general, dental laboratories are set up in a series of stations. Each station is dedicated either to a specific employee or to a specific task. These stations have their own set of tools and most likely a lamp to make the heavily detailed work of a dental laboratory technician easier. These stations may have standard office chairs if the task is most easily performed sitting. Alternatively, there may be no chair if the work requires the employee to stand.

The tools involved in this career are varied. They range from lasers for cutting and sculpting, to machinery that shapes and cuts different materials that are used in the construction of the patient's prosthetics. There are usually a number of computers, which are used to create 3D models of the prosthetics, as well as to calculate different data points needed to effectively create a new dental device.

Because of the machinery and lasers, safety gear like goggles or ear plugs are required when working at these stations. There are also various chemicals and amalgams used as well, which require safe and proper handling, and potentially the use of gloves. This is to protect the employee from potential injury during the prosthetic construction process. Also, because these materials go into the patient's mouth, conditions in a dental laboratory must meet health and sanitation requirements.

A dental laboratory technician may work at only one station, or at a variety of different stations throughout the lab depending on the particular assignment. In some labs, the worker is tasked with performing a single job function in the construction of a prosthetic, while in others, the technician would see each project through from beginning to completion. This primarily depends on the size of the lab staff.

THE WORK YOU WILL DO

DENTAL LABORATORY TECHNICIANS make a significant contribution to oral healthcare by making the products and devices that help improve teeth. These include things like bridges, partial and full dentures, and splints. Dental technicians make these products from a variety of materials including waxes, plastics, precious and non-precious alloys, stainless steel, and a variety of porcelains and composites or polymer glass combinations. Dental techs also use materials such as ceramic and metal, to fabricate porcelain veneers, implants, and crowns used in restorative and cosmetic dentistry.

There are many reasons a patient may need a dental laboratory technician to make a prosthetic piece, including:

Fill in gaps

Improve bite and occlusion

Straighten teeth

Improve teeth function

Prevent future problems that could lead to tooth loss

Enhance the patient's smile through a more uniform shape or color

Promote general dental health

To serve these needs, dental laboratory technicians fill prescriptions from dentists for crowns, bridges, dentures, and other dental prosthetics.

Dentures

To create dentures, for example, the dentist first sends a specification of the item to be fabricated, along with an impression of the patient's mouth or teeth, and written instructions. Then, the dental laboratory technician creates a model of the patient's mouth by pouring plaster or another amalgam into the impression and allowing it to set. Next, the model is placed on an apparatus that mimics the bite and movement of the patient's jaw. The model serves as the basis of the prosthetic device. The technician examines the model, noting the size and shape of the adjacent teeth, as well as gaps within the gum line. The dental tech then sculpts the model according to the mouth dimensions of the individual patient using a variety of tools like lasers and hand-held tools.

Replicating a Tooth

Replicating a single tooth starts the same way. Using the dentist's specifications as well as the technician's own observations, the tech builds and shapes a wax model, using small hand instruments called wax spatulas and wax carvers. The wax model is used to cast the metal framework for the prosthetic device. After the wax tooth has been formed, the technician pours the cast and forms the metal. Using small hand-held tools, he then prepares the surface to allow the metal and porcelain to bond. The porcelain is applied in layers until it arrives at the precise shape and color of a tooth. The tooth is then placed in a porcelain furnace to bake the porcelain onto the metal framework. Any adjustment to the shape and color will be done with subsequent grinding and addition of porcelain to achieve a sealed finish. The final product is nearly an identical replica of the lost tooth.

Making Dental Prosthetics

When creating a new prosthetic, dental laboratory technicians must pay close attention to minute details. They take great care to follow all specifications in the order to ensure that the device will fit properly in the patient's mouth. The work requires skill in the use of sophisticated instruments, equipment, and laboratory procedures. That is the technical part of the job, but there is also an artistic aspect that is equally important. The technician's goal is to make the teeth look as uniform as possible, whether the patient is receiving a crown, veneer, bridge, implant, or dentures. Techs have to anticipate what would look best in the patient's mouth and imagine how the piece fits in where there are no teeth presently. It is important for the technician to create tooth replacements that are both attractive and functional. Even the smallest deviation in shape or size, or a subtle difference in the shade of color can ruin an otherwise perfect smile. The effects of these prosthetics are long lasting, leaving an impression on the patient's life long after the prosthetic is created and delivered to the dentist.

Dental laboratory technicians can specialize in five areas. These areas include ceramics, crowns and bridges, complete dentures, partial dentures, and orthodontics.

Dental technicians who specialize in ceramics will work on constructing things like porcelain veneers for patients who want to fix cosmetic problems with their teeth. These veneers are individual pieces that are adhered to the front of the teeth by the dentist. They can cover stains and uneven textures in the shape of the teeth. They also prevent future staining by protecting the enamel from acid and damage from food and beverages.

Dental laboratory technicians who specialize in crowns and bridges create structures that are used to repair existing teeth. Crowns are caps that go over the top of existing damaged or decayed teeth. A bridge is simply two crowns and one false tooth. It is created to bridge the gap between missing teeth. Dental laboratory technicians make these out of a combination of ceramic crowns and a material that binds the crowns to one another behind the front of the teeth.

Another specialty is complete dentures. These are required when a patient is missing all the teeth. Dentures are artificial teeth that take the place of natural teeth. As this is a full set of new teeth, it is very important that they look uniform in a patient's mouth. This is when an eye for detail becomes crucial.

Partial dentures are a different and separate specialty. Unlike complete dentures, partial dentures are utilized when a patient has some teeth and only requires a few new teeth to replace the missing ones.

The final specialty area, orthodontics, is the art of straightening existing teeth through a device such as traditional metal braces, or Invisalign and retainers. Dental braces are the traditional way of straightening crooked teeth, using metal or ceramic brackets and wires to pressure the teeth into place. Invisalign is a newer, more expensive technology that uses clear, removable aligners. Invisalign is more convenient and aesthetically appealing but dentists prefer braces for certain orthodontic treatments such as cylindrical tooth rotation, vertical movement of teeth, or correcting a significantly large overbite.

Regardless of the product that dental laboratory technicians manufacture, they must follow the regulations set forth by the Food and Drug Administration (FDA). These devices are considered medical devices and they have their own special set of strict regulations in order to protect the patient who receives them.

In some laboratories, technicians perform all stages of the work, while in other labs, each technician does only a few, or even just one. Dental laboratory technicians can specialize in one of five areas: orthodontic appliances, crowns and bridges, complete dentures, partial dentures, or ceramics. Job titles can reflect specialization in these areas. For example, technicians who make porcelain and acrylic restorations are called dental ceramists.

Many dental laboratory technicians will work with a number of dentists depending on how large their laboratory is and how many dentists it serves. One dental technician may represent the patients of several dentists at the same time. These dentists may not even be in the same town as the laboratory. Therefore, the dental laboratory technician might be receiving impressions and instructions from dentists who are many miles or even states away, depending on the geographical area a laboratory serves.

In addition, dental laboratory technicians do some standard office paperwork, including managing inventory reports and preparing laboratory records. The amount of paperwork grows with job advancement. For example, supervisors have many reports to write, while dental laboratory technicians spend most of their time working on the prosthetics.

While this work tends to be more independent, the staff of each laboratory becomes a team. You become familiar with the people working around you, and while you are working on your own project, there is a sense of community. The team also shapes your daily work activities as well. Depending on how the laboratory supervisor divides the workload, you may work on only one part of a prosthetic, or you may be involved in a more complete execution, handling the work from start to finish.

Laboratory Supervisors

Laboratory supervisors manage the dental laboratory technicians, their workload, and the supplies throughout the laboratory. This includes handling personnel disputes, hiring and firing staff, and extending disciplinary action if necessary. Supervisors may also be in charge of promoting staff within the company and doling out performance reviews. Laboratory supervisors often determine who fits best in different roles, and they can have a large say in the sorts of activities a dental laboratory technician performs throughout the day.

They also create systems for efficiency and planning, keeping everyone on task and making sure that the projects are delivered in a timely manner to the customer. Laboratory supervisors also monitor the equipment throughout the lab, managing the repair of anything that might be broken, replacing equipment if necessary and keeping it maintained. Supervisors also do reporting.

Laboratory Owner

Laboratory owners are responsible for running their own businesses. With this comes everything from ordering supplies, to hiring and firing staff, finding the perfect space for the laboratory, staying abreast of the latest technologies to include in the laboratory, keeping track of the numbers and accounting to ensure the laboratory stays profitable.

Owners also represent their laboratories in their communities, handling some of the marketing and the acquisition of new customers. Although different members of the staff can handle each of these duties, it takes a while to build these systems and teams, and the owner will end up doing much of this work.

Educators

Educators may work in a functioning laboratory or in a training facility, such as a local technical college, or in a military capacity. They are in charge of developing new talent in the field, assisting beginners in selecting their specialty, introducing concepts, and testing for people's understanding of the material and techniques. They administer examinations and grade them as well. They also ensure that their students are practicing under the proper regulations set forth by the different regulating bodies in the field. Educators do not have to have direct laboratory experience, but it is helpful in understanding the field and will make for a much better teacher.

Sales

Sales representatives act as the liaisons between the dental laboratory and the dentists it serves. These salespeople go out and acquire new dentists for the laboratory. Orders from these dentists will ultimately earn more income for the laboratory. They build relationships with these dentists and provide customer service throughout the process in case anything goes wrong. Sales representatives are there to grow the reach of the dental laboratory. They may travel to multiple cities to sign on new dentists for the lab. (The other dental laboratory roles do not require travel.)

The reach of the dental laboratory depends on what is wanted by the management and the owner of the laboratory. Some salespeople will be on the road 100 percent of the time, acquiring new work, while others may remain local and will simply go out on sales calls in the nearby community, instead of traveling far and wide. In general, the larger the laboratory, the more salespeople it will use. It is not required that sales representatives have previous experience constructing the devices themselves, but a thorough knowledge of the products is required to sell them effectively. This does not have to come from direct experience in the laboratory, although that can help.

DENTAL LAB TECHNICIANS TELL THEIR OWN STORIES

I Am the Owner of an Independent Dental Laboratory

"Like a lot of high school kids, I didn't know what career path I wanted to take. My uncle was a dentist, and he urged me to consider attending a trade school for dental technicians. I looked into it, but discovered that graduates started out on the job earning about the same salary as non-graduates. This isn't necessarily the case today, but that was 20 years ago. I made the logical choice at the time and found a trainee position. Right from the start, I knew I had found my calling.

My training was very thorough and I became experienced in the various aspects of the job by working in every department of a large lab. It took about a year to complete the training. I was then assigned to the grinding and polishing station, which is the final step in the fabrication process. This role suited me well because I'm a perfectionist. Every device that left my station was smooth and flawless.

After a few years, I became restless and wanted to use more of the skills I had been taught. I took a job as an in-house technician for a dental office. It was a great move. I learned more about the practical side of device manufacturing, and I was exposed to clinical dentistry and the many nuances of patient contact. For the first time, I was able to put a face to the patients that would be wearing teeth I had created. This made a huge difference in how I perceived my work. I had always experienced job satisfaction, but actually seeing the end results takes it to a different level. Problem solving and producing a product that can change a person's quality of life are very rewarding.

I established my own dental lab about five years ago. The technicians I hire have the unusual ability to blend art and science. I look for people who enjoy the creativity that comes with the artistic side of the work, yet embrace the discipline and order of the science behind what they do. In this field, it is important that you enjoy what you do before trying to make a career out of it. If you love sculpting or painting and also enjoy working on computers, this could be a good fit.

Dental technology is developing rapidly and so is the need for dental technicians – particularly those with clinical skills to work with dentists or directly with patients. The best way to get started is to make an appointment to visit and tour a lab. Make sure the owner or manager is going to be present so you can talk about your desire to enter the field. Being proactive like this is the best way to get your foot in the door with an entry-level job.

Be prepared for the low pay starting out with no experience. Keep in mind that as you stick with it and keep gaining more experience, the benefits of the career will continue to grow. Once your knowledge base begins to develop and you have proven yourself, you can make a good living in a field that is very rewarding."

I Am a Dental Ceramist

"I have been a ceramist for 10 years. I did not set out to be in any kind of healthcare field. In fact, I have a degree in fine arts. Like many art school graduates, I found it hard to find a steady job where I could apply my talents. Fortunately, my guidance counselor was married to a dentist. She told me about dental technology and how it's a great fit for artists. I was dubious at first, but I did some research and discovered that she was right.

My job is to create individual teeth for implants. The work starts with an impression of the patient's mouth and a prescription from the dentist. I use the impression as a guide while building up a wax version of the prosthesis. When the wax model fits the impression exactly, I use it to make a form. Then I pour dental ceramic into the form, let it set, and put it in a ceramic kiln. After it's fired, it's cleaned and polished. I refer to photographs to match the natural color of the patient's teeth. Color matching is important to make sure that the prosthesis blends in with the natural teeth.

This is very exacting work. I have to make sure that the prosthetic is the right size and shape for the patient's mouth, while also balancing aesthetic concerns so that the impression does not stand out. That's where a background in art really helps.

There is a lot of opportunity in this field for talented technicians. Talent is the key that opens doors. The field of cosmetic dentistry is growing fast, and so are patients' expectations. It is becoming increasingly difficult for dentists and labs to find competent techs, especially those who can create realistic implants. In many areas, employers have positions open that they can't fill.

If the field interests you at all, don't be deterred by the low starting pay. I started out at minimum wage. Since I was a starving artist, that didn't bother me at all. A year later, I was making $20 an hour. I moved to a bigger city and was immediately bumped up to $30. Today, my salary is close to $40 an hour plus benefits. It's been a very good way to put my art degree to work."

PERSONAL QUALIFICATIONS

IF YOU HAVE A GOOD BALANCE OF love for technology, art, and health, as well as fine motor skills, you would do well as a dental lab technician.

The personal character trait of creativity is an integral part of a career in dental lab technology, because you will be working to recreate a patient's actual smile. This means paying very close attention to detail and noticing things like the shape of the teeth, as well as minute changes in color and shading. In this way, it is like drawing a portrait, except that instead of paint brushes or pencils on canvas, you are using small tools on materials like wax, plastic and alloy. Having a creative eye allows you to translate the details of a person's smile into the prosthetic you are making for them. You can also anticipate changes in a person's smile, and imagine what their ideal appearance would be if they had all their original teeth, because your eye for detail allows you to pull it all together.

Dental laboratory technicians are very skilled with their hands. They use a variety of small tools and lasers to execute designs, and shape and mold the prosthetics they are creating. This involves fine motor skills and dexterity as well as very developed hand-eye coordination.

You should feel comfortable with technology and be able to pick it up quickly. Today's dental lab techs need to be adept at using computer programs, especially those that focus on 3D modeling, because these are frequently the first steps in creating a prosthetic.

In order to excel in the field of dental technology, it is imperative that you be a lifelong learner. That is because new technology is always emerging.

Because of the unique laboratory environment, you should also feel comfortable working both independently and with a team. It is not a social job, in that you do not interface directly with patients, but you will have other team members or dentists who will rely on you to complete your piece of the prosthetic production puzzle. While your work is done independently, you will be accountable to others.

ATTRACTIVE FEATURES

ONE OF THE BIGGEST ATTRACTIONS OF the dental laboratory technician career is the high demand. As cosmetic procedures boom in the modern world, more dental laboratory technicians are needed to manufacture veneers, crowns and dentures that give patients the perfect smile. With the high demand comes a high level of job security. The services performed by dental technicians will always be needed. With the population growing older, there will be a growing demand for prostheses that improve appearance, and the ability to speak clearly and to eat efficiently.

This is a rewarding career. Dental technicians play a significant role in the delivery of a valued healthcare service. The work directly impacts patients' lives, positively affecting people's oral health and self-image. Because of a prosthetic that you have created, they are more comfortable when they chew and feel more confident when they look in the mirror. You can take pride from producing a handcrafted product that will be appreciated for many years to come.

Dental lab technicians also get the chance to test out the latest in technology, making it a fun career choice for early adopters and those who like to work with electronics and machines. As technologies change, so does the equipment in the lab. As equipment is swapped out, there is an opportunity to learn a new skill and test it in real life. It is an ideal working environment for people who consider themselves lifelong learners.

There is also a healthy balance of art and science to be found in this career path, for those who would rather not give up one or the other. Data is collected to determine the shape and features of the prosthetics. They are applied in the creation process, but there is no final product until a touch of creativity is added. The coloring, the shapes, and how it all fits together require the skill and touch of an artist.

Dental laboratory technology is a flexible career, offering several opportunities for advancement. Experienced technicians can find well-paid positions in commercial laboratories based on their technical and communications skills. They can become department heads in larger laboratories where they would have supervisory responsibilities, and they potentially can own their own laboratory. Dental technicians also may teach dental technology courses in educational programs and apply their knowledge to research, sales, and marketing of prosthetic materials, instruments and equipment.

UNATTRACTIVE FEATURES

SOME MAY FIND THE STARTING SALARY for dental laboratory technicians low compared to other starting salaries in the healthcare fields, particularly when compared to dentists. A dental laboratory technician can expect to start out making around $25,000 per year, while dentists can top $100,000 in their first years. The major difference is in the amount of time and training required for the career. Dental laboratory technicians spend much less time in school, accounting for the disparity.

People who prefer to be active and work outdoors will find the dental laboratory technician job unsuitable. If you get restless and struggle to stay in one building, or even one room, for an entire scheduled shift, this may not be the career for you. It is a job that promotes a sedentary lifestyle and the daily routine can become tedious.

Much of the dental tech's work is done independently, but you do have to answer to supervisors and dentists throughout each project. This can be difficult for people who struggle with authority or simply prefer autonomy.

Some may find the creative aspect of the work challenging, especially those who assumed it only required technical skills. You must anticipate what a missing tooth would look like in a patient's mouth, compensating for curves, shape, and color variations on an object you have never seen before. You are essentially creating something out of thin air and that requires a good visual imagination. This is not just a technical job as the name implies, it is also artistry.

A lab technician's eyes, hands, and wrists may get tired or strained from doing such small, detailed tasks over and over again. Back pain from being regularly hunched over is not unusual.

Depending on the tools in the laboratory, there can be some risks to personal health and safety. There are a variety of chemicals and amalgams used in the construction of prosthetics, each of which comes with its own set of safety standards. Machines used for cutting can cause injury in some cases, and lasers can burn skin or eyes if used incorrectly. These risks can be minimized by taking the proper safety precautions.

EDUCATION AND TRAINING

THERE IS MORE THAN ONE WAY TO get the necessary education and training to become a dental laboratory technician. The path you choose depends on what role you would like to have in the field and how far up the standard industry ladder you would like to climb.

The most popular option is to complete a two-year associate degree program in dental technology. You should look for a program accredited by the American Dental Association (ADA). This training can be found in technical schools, community colleges, and the military. An associate degree program in dental technology provides an overview of the field, teaches the specific dental laboratory techniques used today, and equips the graduate with the basic skills needed to advance in the career.

These skills can also be acquired through on-the-job training and apprenticeships. These are paid opportunities – though the pay is lower than that of a fully trained laboratory technician. While these programs do not require previous training to start, openings are not unlimited, and some applicants will not be immediately accepted. Having a proven interest in the field through something like a two-year degree in dental technology can provide a competitive edge.

As a trainee or an apprentice, you would shadow an advanced lab tech, learning about the different tools and technologies, and the methods that particular lab uses for creating prosthetics. The training typically starts with small tasks like pouring plaster into the molds the dentist makes of the patient's teeth. From there, the tasks become more advanced, until the trainee is able to create dentures and crowns.

These programs are designed to take a beginner all the way up to the level of being able to work unsupervised. The National Association for Dental Laboratories keeps a listing of laboratories that offer paid trainee positions.

Dental laboratory technicians can specialize in five different areas. These include ceramics, crowns and bridges, complete dentures, partial dentures, and orthodontics. Choosing a specialty determines what training you will need and what skills you will use in your work. Specialties do not necessarily limit your job opportunities, but they do make it more likely that you will get a job in that particular area.

Certification

The National Board for Certification in Dental Laboratory Technology offers voluntary testing and certification for dental laboratory technicians who want to stand out among the competition in the field. This is not mandatory, but getting certified can potentially lead to greater earnings potential, and you may have an easier time finding jobs.

To become a Certified Dental Technician (CDT), you must have demonstrated the mastery of all five of the specialty areas, as well as a commitment to the field of dental technology. The certification is given upon completion of a formal examination process. Applicants must have never been convicted of practicing illegal dentistry, must possess a mastery of the English language, and have demonstrated ample experience in the field. There are three examinations to take, in any order, and they can be spread out over a four-year period. The three examinations include a written comprehensive exam consisting of 160 multiple-choice questions, a specialty practical and a specialty written examination consisting of 80 multiple-choice questions. Candidates must apply to take this examination.

This certification can be costly especially if you are just starting out in the field and are not earning the income to support it. Two-thirds of those who obtain their certification choose to keep it active for more than 10 years.

Advancement

Courses in business and management are recommended if you are considering working your way up the laboratory ladder, starting as a laboratory technician and advancing to a supervisory or management role. For laboratory supervision, management or ownership, classes in accounting, business, project management, and human resources can be good preparation. This kind of coursework is especially important for those who want to open their own labs. You may want to enroll in a four-year business school to help ensure your success as a business owner.

If it is a career as a dental laboratory technician educator or salesperson that interests you, start with basic training in this field either through an apprenticeship or through an associate degree. From there, supporting classes in education and classroom instruction can help prepare you for a degree in teaching. Aspiring sales reps may want to take classes in advertising and marketing to learn the art of selling. This can also be accomplished by taking an entry-level sales job and transitioning into the dental laboratory world.

EARNINGS

THE ANNUAL SALARY FOR A DENTAL laboratory technician depends on your specific job role, location, and skills.

On average, dental laboratory technicians start at $25,000 a year and can reach $50,000 after training is completed. The nationwide average is $45,000. Technicians in large laboratories tend to specialize in a few procedures and are typically paid a lower wage than those employed in small laboratories that perform a variety of tasks. Those located in big urban areas are paid considerably more than those in small towns.

Some technicians are paid hourly and others are salaried. Those who are paid hourly wages are only paid for the exact number of hours a week they work. Therefore, annual income is dependent on the total number of hours worked. Salaried jobs are paid the same amount annually regardless of how many hours the employee spends in the lab. Salaries are often seemingly higher than hourly wages, but that may not end up being the case if days run longer than usual, since you will not receive overtime pay.

Salaried jobs do have the advantage of providing benefits – something hourly wage earners may not receive. Salaried technicians usually enjoy compensation packages that include health insurance, paid sick leave, retirement plans, and paid vacation days. Two weeks of paid vacation is standard in the dental field.

Experienced and skilled dental laboratory technicians who want to earn more usually do so by becoming a dental laboratory supervisor or a dental laboratory owner. Supervisors earn on average about $20,000 more than staff technicians. Business owners earn even more. Their potential income is limited only by how big they want to grow their companies.

Dental laboratory technology educators are paid based on their experience and location. Some might be employed by the laboratories themselves to train new hires, while others work for a local training program or technical college.

For dental laboratory technicians who work in sales, there are two different structures for earnings. In the first scenario, a salesperson in this field would earn an annual salary or base pay not dependent on how many new dentists are signed up with the lab. In an alternative arrangement, income would be based entirely on commissions earned. This is either a percentage of the total amount of sales brought into the lab, or a set referral fee based on the number of new clients. These commissions may or may not be capped. There are often incentive bonuses offered for meeting sales goals. Ambitious dental sales reps can earn as much as $100,000 a year.

OPPORTUNITIES

WITH DEVELOPMENTS LIKE MAKEOVER TV shows, baby boomers wanting to look younger, selfie culture, and celebrity obsessions, physical appearance is taking a front seat in many people's lives. As a society, we are beginning to prioritize how we look – and we are not shy about spending money to look better. This goes beyond the clothing we pick out, the jewelry we wear, and the way we style our hair – it is reaching us on a more fundamental level. Many are now changing their very physical structures, making cosmetic dentistry the biggest area of dental laboratory technology growth.

As the general population becomes more interested in cosmetic procedures, including cosmetic dentistry, the demand for dental laboratory technicians will be greater than ever. New jobs are being created to fill this demand. Cosmetic dentistry, together with the devices that allow for perfect teeth, is anticipated to become a $13 billion industry in the coming years. This industry growth will lead to the opening of new labs and the expansion of existing labs, which translates into the creation of new jobs.

As baby boomers age, the many years of bad habits like smoking and drinking are beginning to take a toll on their teeth. This means that the enamel is beginning to decay, causing cavities, fissures, and cracks. In certain situations, an extraction, the removal of the tooth, might also be necessary, leaving an open spot in the gums. In cases such as these, fillings, crowns, or partial dentures may be needed. That means more work for highly trained dental laboratory technicians.

Because dental laboratory techs are in greater demand, there is also a greater demand for people to train them.

This means that the area of education is also set to experience additional growth over the next five years as more teachers are needed to offer training, create curriculum, and lead the next generation of dental laboratory techs to their new careers in the industry.

A study by the American Academy of Dentistry found that dentists are becoming increasingly loyal to the laboratories they use, up almost 60 percent from previous years. Loyalty between dentists and dental laboratories eliminates price comparison shopping, and indicates the chance for dental laboratory technicians to form longer-term relationships with the dentists and the patients they serve. This situation creates greater job security for those already employed, but unless the laboratory is making a concerted effort to expand its client base, it tends to reduce the number of openings for beginners.

GETTING STARTED

THERE ARE A FEW DIFFERENT WAYS TO land your first job as a dental laboratory technician. First, you can graduate from a two-year program and leverage that experience as well as your relationships with your teachers to get started in the industry. Your teachers are an excellent resource for job searching since many of them worked in the profession themselves before becoming a teacher, and in some cases they still are. They will have industry contacts that they can share with you.

To be a standout candidate, it is important to truly apply yourself during school, achieving good grades and making an extra effort to get to know the teachers. Remember that your teachers will only be willing to put their reputations on the line and make introductions on your behalf if you have proven that you are committed to doing your best in this career.

Your school will also have a career guidance office. There you will find information on job fairs and postings of job openings. You can also get advice and help with résumé writing and developing strong interviewing skills.

Be proactive and arrange informational interviews with a local dental laboratory technician, dental laboratory technician supervisor, or dental laboratory technician owner. They will have direct industry knowledge and can give you the answers to the questions you have about working in the field. Come prepared for these meetings in proper attire just as you would to attend a job interview. Informational interviews do not always lead to job offers, so do not be disappointed if you walk out of your meeting without an offer in hand. In fact, it is best to go not expecting a job offer at all. Instead, be genuinely interested in what the person has to say. Be prepared with specific questions you want answered. Usually people are happy to help, especially if you demonstrate that you are enthusiastic about your new career path.

Look for the local chapter of the National Board for Certification in Dental Laboratory Technology. Getting involved locally is a great way to introduce yourself to potential employers who can offer advice and tips as well as potential job opportunities. This organization presents job fairs and networking events where you can meet laboratory owners who are in a position to offer jobs.

Many laboratories also offer trainee positions. Contact laboratories directly by visiting their websites and scanning their career opportunities page, or simply call to inquire about potential job openings. In general, it is best to have an introduction before you send your résumé to someone new.

ASSOCIATIONS

■ **National Association of Dental Laboratories**
https://nadl.org/home-page.cfm

■ **National Board for Certification in Dental Laboratory Technology**
http://www.nbccert.org

■ **The American Dental Association (ADA)**
www.ada.org

■ **Commission on Dental Accreditation**
http://www.ada.org/en/home-ada/coda

PERIODICALS

■ **Lab Management Today**
http://lmtmag.com

■ **Dental Products Report**
www.dentalproductsreport.com/lab

■ **Chairside**
http://www.glidewelldental.com/dentist/chairside

WEBSITES

■ **I Hire Dental**

www.ihiredental.com/t-Dental-Lab-Technician-jobs.html

■ **Bates Technical College**

http://www.bates.ctc.edu/DentalLab

■ **McFatter Technical Center**

http://www.mcfattertech.com

■ **The Dawson Academy**

http://thedawsonacademy.com

/main-navigation/find-a-course/for-lab-techs

■ **Portland Community College**

http://www.pcc.edu/programs/dental-tech/

■ **Durham Technical Community College**

http://www.durhamtech.edu/health

/dentallabtechnology.htm

■ **AmeriTech College**

http://www.ameritech.edu/DentalLaboratoryTechnician

■ **Atlanta Technical College**

http://www.atlantatech.edu/academics/area.php?area

=Dental+Laboratory+Technology